DANDELION

MARIAN KIM

ISBN: 1508575037

ISBN-13: 978-1508575030

CONTENTS

1

PROPERTIES

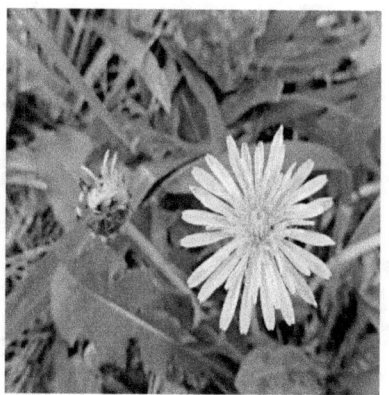

Scientific name: Taraxacum officinale

Other names: Blowball, cankerwort, lion's tooth, swine snout

Nutrients: Dandelion leaves or greens contain vitamin A, B1 (thiamine), B2 (riboflavin), B6 (pyridoxine), B9 (folic acid) and C. It also contains minerals like calcium, potassium, iron, magnesium, manganese and zinc. Dandelions also contain fiber.

Properties

Antibacterial properties

Antioxidant properties which protect the cells from free radical damage that causes premature aging and degenerative diseases

Astringent properties

Diuretic (increase urine production) properties

Detoxifying properties

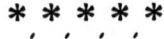

2

USES

Liver disease treatment

Dandelion has been used for centuries to treat jaundice or the yellowing of the skin and eyes that develops as a result of liver disease.

Scurvy treatment

Dandelion decoction is taken for scurvy since it is a very good source of vitamin C.

Eczema treatment

Dandelion decoction is taken for eczema.

Dyspepsia treatment

Dandelion tea is taken for dyspepsia with constipation.

Antipyretic

Dandelion tea is taken for fever.

Insomnia treatment

Dandelion tea is taken for insomnia.

Constipation

Dandelion is used as mild laxative for constipation.

Minor wounds

Dandelion juice is applied on wounds because of its antibacterial action to prevent infections.

Boils and abscess

Dandelion poultices can be applied to boils and abscesses to aid with the healing process.

Tonsillitis relief

Dandelion soup was shown in a study to help patients who had their tonsils removed recover faster when compared to those who drunk soup without dandelion.

Acne treatment

Dandelion is used for acne treatment because of its antibacterial properties. The root is also used to clear rashes.

Joint pain relief

Dandelion is used to manage joint pains. Dandelion infused oils or dandelion salves can be used to relieve the aches.

Weight loss

Dandelions are useful for weight loss because they are rich in fiber and make a person feel fuller for longer. They are thus able to reduce snacking between meals. Dandelions are also natural diuretics. This means they make a person pass urine more frequently and this may also contribute to weight loss.

Digestive aid

Dandelion is used to improve digestion by increasing bile production.

Flatulence relief

Dandelion can be used to relieve flatulence (intestinal gas).

Anorexia relief

Dandelion is used to manage anorexia since it improves the appetite.

Water retention

Dandelions are natural diuretics. This means they make a person pass urine more frequently and are used for water retention. They are also used for urine infections to increase urine flow. They do not deplete potassium levels like some of the synthetic diuretics.

Urinary tract infection (UTI) prevention

Dandelion extracts when combined with those of uva ursi reduce the number of UTIs in women because of their diuretic and antibacterial properties respectively.

Detoxification

Dandelion is used to detoxify the liver and reduce the side effects of prescription medications.

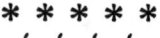

3

SAFETY PRECAUTIONS

1. Person who are allergic to aster family plants like daisies, ragweed, marigolds and chrysanthemums should avoid dandelions.

2. Persons with inflamed or infected gallbladders or blocked bile ducts should not use dandelion.

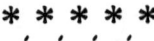

4

DRUG INTERACTIONS

1. Dandelions can adversely interact with antibiotics and reduce how much the body absorbs them as well as their effectiveness. Examples of such antibiotics include ciprofloxacin (Cipro) and norfloxacin (Noroxin).

2. Dandelions can adversely interact with lithium because of its diuretic action. It can increase lithium levels in the body and lead to increased side effects.

3. Dandelion can adversely interact with medications broken down by the liver. It can lead to increased side effects. Examples of such mediations include amitriptyline (Elavil), propranolol (Inderal) and verapamil (Calan).

4. Dandelion can adversely interact with medications that are changed in the liver and decrease their effectiveness. Examples of such mediations include acetaminophen, diazepam (Valium) and digoxin.

5. Dandelions can interact with diuretics or water pills like amiloride (Midamor) and spironolactone (Aldactone) and lead to high levels of potassium in the body.

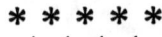

6

HERBAL RECIPES

Dandelion Tea

Equipment

Kettle

Tea cup

***

Ingredients

1 teaspoon of minced dandelion

1 cup of boiling water

Honey to taste (optional)

***

Instructions

1. Put the dandelion in a tea cup, add the boiling water and let it steep while covered for 10 -15 minutes.

2. Add honey (if using) to suit your taste before drinking.

*****

Dandelion Syrup

Equipment

Saucepan

Jar with airtight lid

***

Ingredients

1 quart (1000 ml) filtered water

1 cup dried dandelion or 3 cups fresh dandelion

1 cup honey

***

Instructions

1. Place the water and dandelion in a saucepan and bring to a boil.

2. Reduce the heat and let it simmer while it is partially covered until the volume is reduced to half the original volume.

3. Strain the mixture through a sieve or cheesecloth to remove the dandelion.

4. Measure 1 pint (500 mls) of the liquid and add the honey.

5. Cook for a few minutes as you stir it so that it thickens.

6. Store the syrup in an airtight container in the fridge for up to 2 months.

*****

Dandelion Decoction

Equipment
Non-reactive heavy saucepan

***

Ingredients
1 oz (30 grams) dandelion root powder

1 pint (500 ml) water

***

Instructions
1. Place the dandelion and water in the saucepan, cover them and slowly bring the mixture to a simmering boil for 20 minutes.

2. Remove from the heat source and let the mixture cool to drinking temperature.

3. Strain the mixture, measure it and pour the liquid into a clean saucepan.

4. Heat the liquid until it begins to steam. Reduce the heat and let the liquid continue to steam until it is reduced to half its original volume. This may take 45 minutes to 1 hour.

5. Pour the decoction into a clean bottle.

6. Store the decoction in the refrigerator to lengthen its life.

*****

Dandelion Tincture

Equipment

Glass jar with tight fitting lid

Dark tincture bottles

Cheesecloth

Labels

*

Ingredients

7 oz (200 gm) of dried dandelion or 14 oz (400 gm) of fresh dandelion

30 oz (1 liter) of 80-100 proof vodka

*

Instructions

1. Fill 1/3 of the glass jar with the chopped dandelion.

2. Add the vodka to completely fill the jar to the top.

3. Seal the jar and label it with the date of preparation and name of dandelion used. Store the glass jar in a dark place for 6 weeks ensuring that you shake them weekly.

5. After 6 weeks strain out the dandelion with a cheesecloth and pour the tincture into dark tincture bottles.

6. Label the tincture bottles and store your herbal tinctures away from light and heat.

**

Dandelion Poultice

Equipment

Cheesecloth or old cotton sheet strips

***

Ingredients

1 tablespoon powdered dandelion root

Boiling water

***

Instructions

1. Add enough boiling water to the dandelion to wet it and make a thick paste.

2. Spoon the dandelion paste onto the cheesecloth (or bed sheet strips) to make the poultice.

3. To use, apply the poultice to the affected area and cover with another piece of hot, wet cloth. Replace the hot, wet cloth when it cools with another hot one to keep the poultice hot.

*****

Dandelion Infused Oil

Equipment
Double boiler

Large glass bowl

Sieve and cheesecloth

Sterilized dark jars

***

Ingredients
16 fl oz. (500 ml) vegetable oil like olive or sweet almond oil

8 oz. (250 grams) slightly crushed, dry dandelion or 16 oz. (500 grams) slightly bruised fresh dandelion

***

Instructions
1. Place the dandelion and oil in the glass bowl ensuring that the oil covers the dandelion. Simmer them in a double boiler for 1 hour at around 120 degrees Fahrenheit (49 degrees Celsius). Do not let the mixture boil. You can repeat this step after letting the oils cool to create more concentrated herb infused oils.

2. Strain the mixture through the sieve and cheesecloth into a clean, dark jar ensuring you squeeze out as much oil as you can from the cheesecloth.

3. Label your jars and store your dandelion infused oils in a cool dark place or in the refrigerator and use them within 3 months.

*****

Dandelion Salve

Equipment

Double boiler

Large glass bowl

Sterilized dark jars or tins

***

Ingredients

8 oz. (250 ml or 1 cup) dandelion infused vegetable oil (see previous recipe)

1 oz. (30 grams) beeswax

10 drops essential oils like lavender essential oil (optional natural fragrance)

***

Instructions

1. Place the beeswax and dandelion infused oil in the glass bowl and melt them in a double boiler.

2. Once melted remove from the heat source, allow to cool and add the essential oils (if using).

3. Pour the melted oils into the storage jars or tins and allow to cool completely.

4. Store the salves in a cool dark place.

###

ABOUT THE AUTHOR

Marian Kim is an experienced alternative medicine practitioner.

OTHER BOOKS BY THE AUTHOR

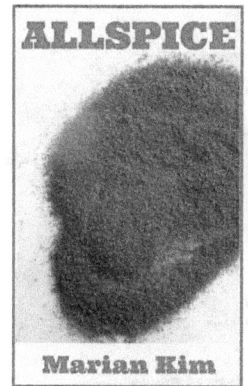

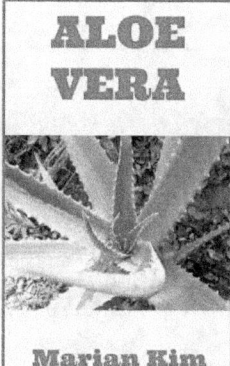

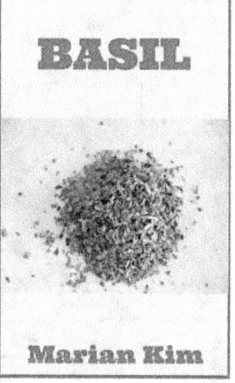

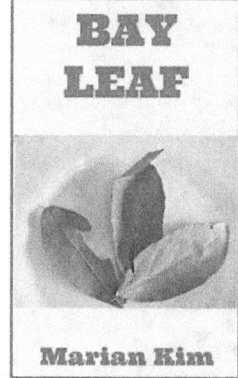

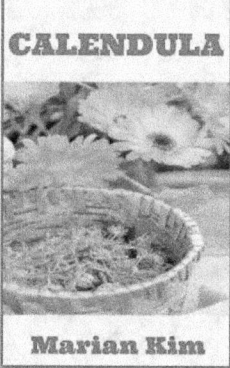

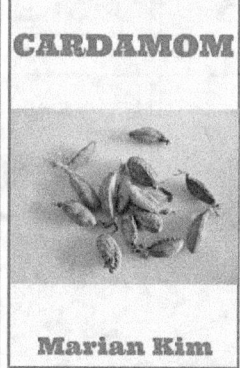

CAYENNE PEPPER
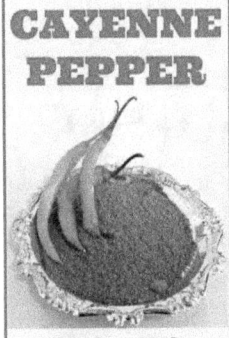
Marian Kim

CHAMOMILE
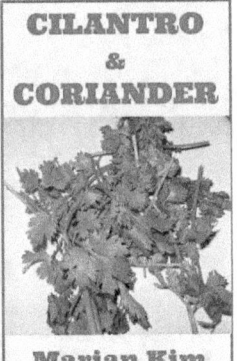
Marian Kim

CILANTRO & CORIANDER
Marian Kim

CINNAMON
Marian Kim

CLOVES
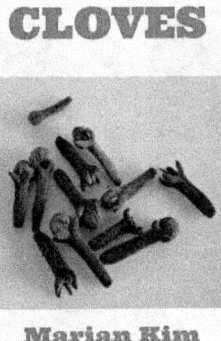
Marian Kim

CUMIN
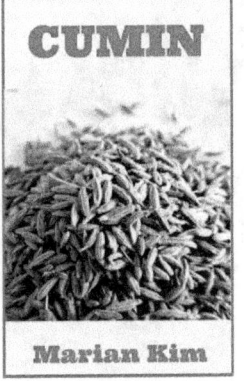
Marian Kim

DANDELION
Marian Kim

DILL
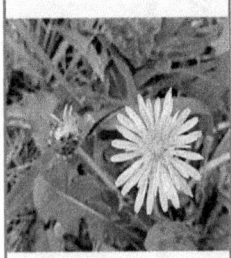
Marian Kim

ECHINACEA
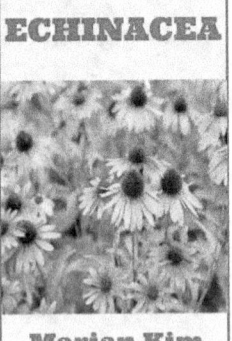
Marian Kim

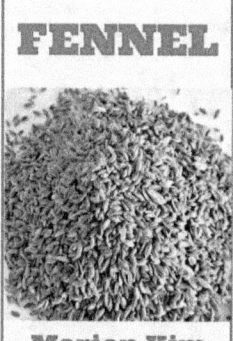

FENNEL

Marian Kim

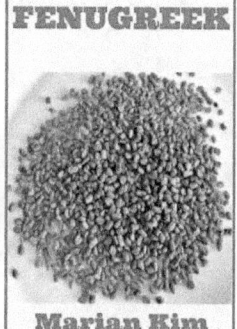

FENUGREEK

Marian Kim

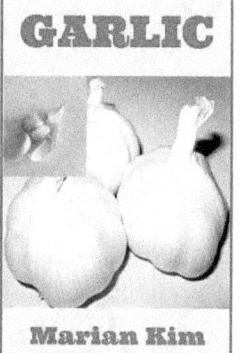

GARLIC

Marian Kim

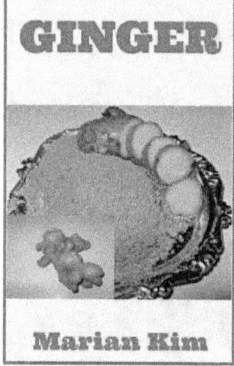

GINGER

Marian Kim

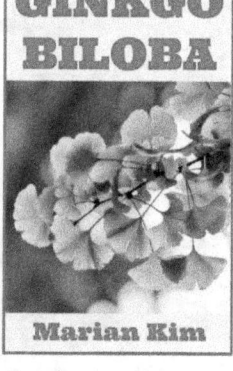

GINKGO BILOBA

Marian Kim

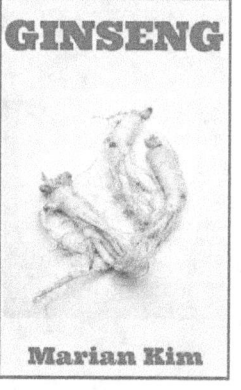

GINSENG

Marian Kim

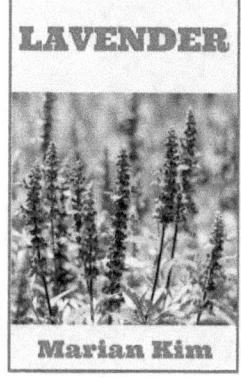

LAVENDER

Marian Kim

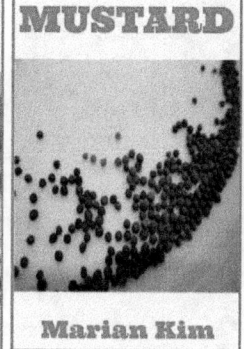

MUSTARD

Marian Kim

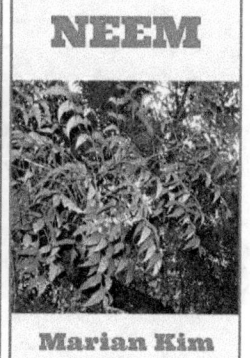

NEEM

Marian Kim

NUTMEG & MACE

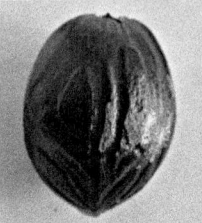

Marian Kim

OREGANO

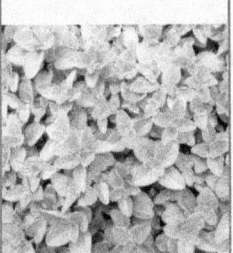

Marian Kim

PAPRIKA

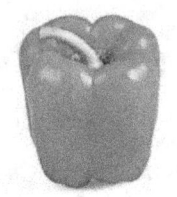

Marian Kim

PARSLEY

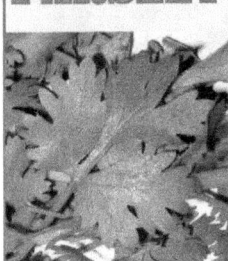

Marian Kim

BLACK & WHITE PEPPER

Marian Kim

PEPPERMINT

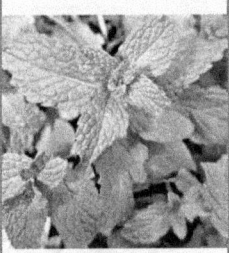

Marian Kim

ROSE HIPS

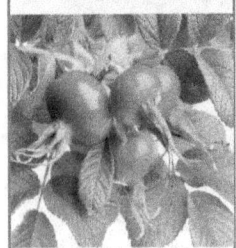

Marian Kim

ROSE PETALS

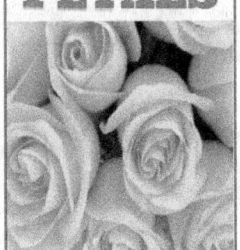

Marian Kim

ROSEMARY

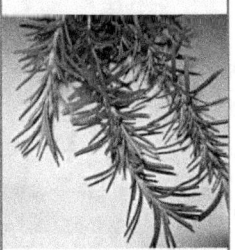

Marian Kim

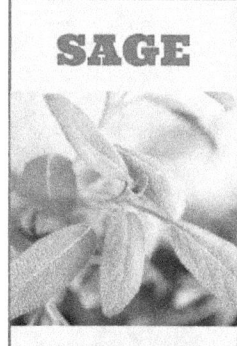

SAGE

Marian Kim

ST. JOHN'S WORT

Marian Kim

STAR ANISE

Marian Kim

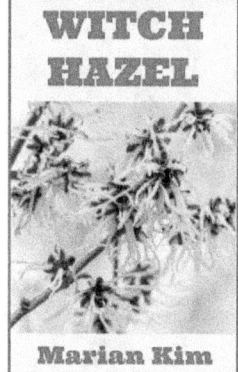

STINGING NETTLE

Marian Kim

THYME

Marian Kim

TURMERIC

Marian Kim

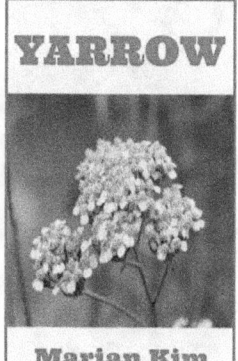

WITCH HAZEL

Marian Kim

YARROW

Marian Kim

*****